Tietze's Syndrome: Causes, Tests and Treatments

Tietze's Syndrome: Causes, Tests and Treatments. Copyright © 2009 by Stephanie Kenrose. All rights reserved.

ISBN 9781449591014

Contents

Chapter One: Introduction 5

Chapter Two: Symptoms 13

Chapter Three: Tietze's Syndrome Causes 17

Chapter Four: Tests 25

Chapter Five: Treatment 29

Chapter Six: Diet 37

Chapter Seven: Selected Recipes 45

Appendix 1 91

References: 95

Chapter One: Introduction

In 1992, I had never heard of Tietze's syndrome. If you'd have asked me what it was, I might have said it had something to do with mosquitoes (Tietze's syndrome is sometimes confused with the sleeping sickness caused by the tsetse fly and referred to incorrectly as *tsetse's syndrome*).

In the spring of 1992, I was taken to the ER with symptoms of a heart attack. I was 26 years old. A crushing feeling enveloped my chest like an elephant was sitting on top of me; the pain was like nothing I had ever experienced. The panic that accompanied the pain was overwhelming--luckily, it wasn't a heart attack, but I left the ER that evening without knowing the cause of my pain. Months later, I still didn't have a diagnosis.

"There's nothing wrong with you," an impatient chest specialist told me after two months of trying to diagnose the excruciating pain in my chest. I'd had tests for heart problems, blood disorders, stomach disorders…all to no avail. "You should consider seeing a psychiatrist," he told me. I took him up on it, briefly, but a year later, I still had the pain (and a prescription for Valium).

The large amounts of ibuprofen I was consuming daily caused acid reflux that burned by esophagus and added more pain to my chest area. I went to a different doctor to ask him for prescription strength Zantac. I was a new patient, so he performed a thorough exam, listening to me as I asked him not to tap my chest. "Where does it hurt?" he asked. I pointed to my ribs. "Everywhere." He tapped my costal cartilage gently. "Here?" he asked. I nodded. "You've got Tietze's Syndrome," he said.

I'd never heard of it. The doctor explained that he'd only heard of it in passing (he was fresh out of medical school), and that all he knew about it was that it was a rare disorder, characterized by crushing pain when the chest is pressed on. Tietze's syndrome, he explained, was like costochondritis; only unlike costochondritis, with Tietze's syndrome the rib cartilage swells and the condition can be chronic--sometimes lasting decades.

Tietze's syndrome was named after a German surgeon named Alexander Tietze (1864-1927), who discovered the disease in 1921. The physician studied at Breslau (Wroclaw), obtaining his doctorate in 1887 and eventually practicing at the Allerheiligen-Hospital. He wrote an excellent textbook on emergency surgery which was published in 1927, and he contributed numerous papers on surgical topics. Ninety years after its discovery, the rare disorder named after him has had only a few hundred cases reported in the medical literature worldwide.

Many sources of information will tell you that Tietze's syndrome is the same as costochondritis. On the contrary, the two conditions are different.

Tietze's syndrome is characterized by inflammation and swelling in the costochondral (rib) cartilage, which causes pain that varies from very mild to so severe that it can mimic a heart attack. Costochondritis and Tietze's syndrome affect the same region of the chest--the cartilage that connects the ribs to the breast bone—but that's about where the similarity ends.

- Tietze's causes inflammation, tenderness, and swelling. According to the Mayo clinic, swelling is absent with costochondritis. Note that you may not be able to feel the swelling—for example, if the Tietze's syndrome is affecting the first costal joint, it may be hidden behind your clavicle.

- Tietze's syndrome affects men and women equally, but according to Wright's Radiology of the Chest and Related Conditions, Tietze's syndrome usually occurs in the 20-40 year-old age range bracket. On the other hand, costochondritis tends to affect women over the age of 40, although anyone can get it. One case highlighted in the literature tells of a two-year-old boy who had a painful swelling in one of his left ribs that was diagnosed as Tietze's syndrome: luckily for the boy, the swelling died down after a few weeks.

- According to *Harrison's Rheumatology,* costochondritis affects the third, fourth, or fifth joints down in between the breast bone and ribs (you can feel these joints with your fingers). Tietze's syndrome tends to affect only one joint in 80% of cases, although the pain may radiate out, making it nearly impossible for a sufferer to tell which rib is causing the pain.

- Costochondritis is usually short-lived, whereas Tietze's syndrome can last for years, turning into a chronic condition. One half of Tietze's syndrome patients have pain that lasts more than one year.

My doctor prescribed Vioxx, which I took for nine months to alleviate the pain. The drug worked wonders, but thankfully I was not one of the estimated 100,000 people who suffered a heart attack due to Vioxx!

That is how my year-long journey into understanding Tietze's syndrome happened. I wasn't crazy or stressed: I had a legitimate disease. Two decades later, I still have Tietze's syndrome, but I've learned ways to manage it.

The fact that it took a full year for doctors to diagnose my condition is no longer puzzling to me. Tietze's syndrome is a rare condition (there are only a few hundred reported cases in the medical literature going back to 1921), and Tietze's syndrome is often confused with other disorders of the chest--even by physicians. These include costochondritis and slipping rib syndrome—which occurs when one of the ribs slips out of place, stretching the ligaments. In Tietze's syndrome, a rib does not slip out of place: the rib stays in place but the costal cartilage swells.

Tietze's syndrome is sometimes confused with costosternal chondrodynia but the two conditions are exact opposites! Costosternal Chondrodynia often affects several ribs. It rarely affects the second costal joint. Some researchers note that most cases of Tietze's syndrome occur *only* in the second costal joint. There are only a few similarities between Tietze's syndrome and Costosternal Chondrodynia: an unknown origin of the disease, the disease's benign (not harmful) nature, and the fact that both disease can last for years.

You may also find Tietze's syndrome called many other names—it may be impossible for you to figure out which disease you have unless you have a diagnostic (such as an ultrasound) performed. Some other names that Tietze's might be called (or mistaken for!):

- Chest wall Syndrome

- Condropathia Tuberosa

- Costal chondritis (same as costochondritis)

- Costochondrial junction syndrome

- Costochondritis

- Cyriax's syndrome (slipping rib syndrome)

- Parasternal chondrodnia

- Peristernal perichondritis

- Thoracochondralgia

- Tsetse Disease

- Tietze's Disease

- Xiphoidalgia

Tietze's syndrome was a frustrating disease in the beginning; if only I had had a correct diagnosis, so much stress and anguish would have been avoided! Understanding what this disease is—and what it isn't—is the first step to effective treatment.

Chapter Two: Symptoms

Doctors are well educated. However, Tietze's syndrome is so rare that even your doctor might miss the diagnosis (he's going to be trying to decide between about three dozen different possibilities for your pain, and Tietze's is way down on that list). Two general practitioners and two specialists missed my diagnosis of Tietze's syndrome; it took one year for me to finally get diagnosed--and that diagnosis made it a lot easier to deal with. This chapter will show you how to tell if you have Tietze's syndrome--a benign inflammation of the ribs--or something more sinister, like Pleomorphic T-cell lymphoma, a rare cancer.

Before continuing, make absolutely sure that your physician has ruled out pain caused by heart problems or other serious illness.

Tietze's Syndrome Symptom Checklist

- Do you have intense pain in the rib cartilage area? That's at the junction between your sternum and ribs. The pain could be so severe you might even mistake it for a heart attack. The pain may radiate, and you may not even be sure of the central location for the pain-- just that it's somewhere in or on your chest.

- Do you have pain in the chest area when rolling over in bed, or trying to get out of bed? This is caused by pressure from the ribs squeezing the inflamed breast plate cartilage. You might feel this pain when otherwise twisting, turning or bending.

- Does the pain radiate from the chest to the arms and shoulders? (The pain might be so severe it could feel like it is coming from everywhere).

- Is the pain worse when breathing? Sometimes even a little movement of the rib cage will cause intense pain.

- Lightly press down on the cartilage area between your sternum (breast plate) and ribs. Is it tender and painful in at least one of the first three ribs?

These questions are the most common about Tietze's and cosotchondritis. The hallmark for Tietze's syndrome is that in addition to the pain described above, usually only one rib is affected--the second or third rib down. There are rare exceptions--for example, if the swelling is in the first joint, it may be hidden under your clavicle and you won't be able to feel the swelling. Feel the connections around your other ribs to see what's normal for you. If you feel swelling at the first, second, or third junctions, you most probably have Tietze's syndrome. However, make sure you see a doctor: there are a couple of cancers that can cause one costal junction to be swollen and painful; skin cancer that has invaded the chest area and Pleomorphic T-cell lymphoma is one example.

The chances of a tumor causing your pain are about as slim as contracting Tietze's syndrome itself (only a few hundred cases have ever been documented in the medical literature). However, the same tests that check for Tietze's syndrome (an MRI or CT-scan) will also be able to definitively tell if you have a tumor.

Tietze's syndrome (unlike cosotchondritis) can turn into a chronic condition lasting years, or even decades. Why should you get a diagnosis instead of waiting for the pain to go away? If your doctor tells you that you have "costochondritis," you might expect the pain to disappear in a few weeks. If it doesn't, you should insist on a test to rule out other causes.

Chapter Three: Tietze's Syndrome Causes

I am fairly certain that a virus caused my Tietze's syndrome. How do I know this? Not because of any body of literature, but because of a bizarre series of coincidences that started with a trip to Ireland and ended with karmic retribution and a divorce.

In February, 1992, I traveled to Ireland on a ferry from Hollyhead to Dublin, a wave-riding roller coaster that took a nauseating two hours. I was on my way to a dog show, with a fellow dog breeder named Gwen. We knew each other from dog shows we attended every few weeks, and shared a love for Siberian huskies, so we had a lot to talk about. Six weeks after I returned home from the trip, I was sitting on a friend's couch watching Star Trek: The Next Generation when a crushing pain enveloped my chest. My friend must have seen my pale face, because she asked "Are you OK?" I wasn't okay. I was in so much pain, I could hardly speak. I've given birth *naturally*, and childbirth paled in comparison to the searing pain I was experiencing in my chest. My friend rushed me to the ER, and I had the sickening, strange feeling that I was not going to make it out of the ER. After I described my symptoms (crushing chest pain), I had a heart-attack work up, and ex-ray to check for blood clots, and finally, after the major tests were negative, a dose of Valium that rendered me stupid enough to actually enjoy shopping at Wal Mart on the way home (driven there by my friend of course).

I took six weeks off of work. Sometime around week five, my ex-husband, John came down with the disease and I began to suspect a virus. The final clue to the origin of my disease came about six months later; I realized that I hadn't seen Gwen (the lady who had accompanied me to Ireland) in many months. In fact, no one had seen nor heard of her since the Ireland trip. I called her on the phone and asked her if she had any plans to go to any dog shows in the near future. She said no. "I came down with a disease," she said. "I'm in so much pain…I can't do anything."

After speaking to Gwen on the phone, I discovered we had the same ailment. And like me, she had come down with it a few weeks after our return from Ireland. Add that to my ex-husband coming down with the disorder six weeks after I returned home, and we had out answer: our ailment was caused by a virus.

Although researchers have yet to figure out all of the causes of Tietze's Syndrome, they have some pretty good ideas, from as benign as coughing to as frightening as cancer. More than one of the following conditions in combination may cause Tietze's Syndrome and it's often hard or even impossible to pinpoint an exact cause.

- *Trauma, Recurrent Microtrauma, or Intercostal hematoma.* A fast, unexpected movement could cause a pool of blood—a bruise—to form in the costal cartilage. Bruises (hematomas) in the cartilage joining the ribs to the breast bone (the intercostal area) have been seen in baseball players, but it could be cause by something unexpected like shaking a rug.

- Recurrent episodes of micro trauma to the chest wall: boxing, karate and other martial arts, severe vomiting and/or coughing, are examples of where the chest could experience continuous trauma, but it could be as simple as lifting heavy objects in an awkward fashion over time.

  - *Fibromyalgia.* Fibromyalgia is a chronic, disabling disorder that occurs in about 2% of the population, and is seen more in women that in men. The cause of fibromyalgia is not known, but significantly higher levels of substance P (a neurotransmitter responsible for transmitting pain signals) have been found in the spinal fluid of patients with fibromyalgia. The inflamed costochondral margins that are commonly associated with Tietze's syndrome are the same as two of the pressure points associated with fibromyalgia; it's therefore important that all of a patient's symptoms are taken into account when making a diagnosis of Tietze's.

- *Arthritis and related diseases.* Rarely, patients with psoriatic arthritis have reported Tietze's syndrome; psoriatic arthritis is a condition where arthritis is accompanied by red patches of inflamed skin. Other arthritis related diseases (i.e. ankylosing spondylitis, reactive arthritis and Reiter's disease) might also produce Tietze's syndrome.

- *Ulcerative colitis or Crohn's disease.* Patients with inflammatory bowel disease such as ulcerative colitis and Crohn's disease often report costochondritis and Tietze's syndrome.

- *Cancer.* An Italian study led by R. Cocco found that several patients who were diagnosed with

Tietze's syndrome actually had tumors. The patients all had the classic signs of Tietze's syndrome—swelling of the costal cartilage, pain--and they were all treated with a standard treatment for the disease: anti-inflammatory drugs and an injection of cortisol. When symptoms didn't improve, the patients sought answers: three of the cases were later found to have Hodgkin's disease and one person had non-Hodgkin's lymphoma. All four patients made a complete recovery after the cancer was diagnosed.

- *Heredity factors.* No one knows exactly what causes Tietze's syndrome, but it's thought there could certainly be a hereditary factor. It could run in families—perhaps because of a genetic abnormality.

- *Radiation Therapy.* If you have had radiation therapy to the chest or breast area, there is a chance you will experience Tietze's syndrome sometime down the road (it could be years after the therapy).

- *Syphilis.* Some studies of Tietze's syndrome have linked syphilis to outbreaks of Tietze's syndrome.

- *Stress.* There's no definitive research to suggest that stress causes Tietze's syndrome, but it can make an underlying condition like fibromyalgia worse.

- *Viruses.* A virus caused my Tietze's syndrome; could it have caused yours?

Tietze's syndrome is a rare disease by itself. However, there are a few unusual cases of Tietze's syndrome reported in the medical journals. It's unlikely that your Tietze's syndrome is caused by one of these very rare occurrences.

- Breast Implants. One breast cancer survivor who had reconstructive surgery (with large breast implants) ended up suffering from Tietze's syndrome due to the large implants rubbing against her ribs.

- *Skin Cancer.* One unfortunate patient, diagnosed with Tietze's syndrome, found out that although his symptoms were identical to Tietze's syndrome, further diagnostics revealed he actually had skin cancer which had invaded his inner chest.

- *Malignant Tumor.* There's at least one person out there who is glad he didn't accept a diagnosis of Tietze's syndrome. One patient presented with typical symptoms of Tietze's syndrome--pain in one left costal cartilage. After a biopsy, it was revealed he had Pleomorphic T-cell lymphoma: cancer. While an MRI or CT scan could have caught the tumor, X-rays could not.

- *E-Coli.* One case of E-coli in a diabetic woman led to a severe case of costochondritis. Although different, Tietze's syndrome is closely related to costochondritis, so it isn't so farfetched to think that E-Coli could occasionally cause the disease.

Chapter Four: Tests

There are several tests that can be undertaken to determine whether you have Tietze's syndrome or not. Why test? Because testing can aid you with treating your disease and will rule out other causes, like fibromyalgia and cancer. Your doctor may recommend one of the following techniques to rule out other disorders:

- *Computed tomography* (sometimes known as a CT or CAT scan) is one of the most exact ways to diagnose Tietze's syndrome.

- *Xeroradiography* (a technique commonly used for mammograms) allows a doctor to see a complete picture of the chest wall and rule out other cause of your pain, such as tumors.

- Ultrasound. Researchers Kamel and Kotob report that ultrasound should be the "first choice" screening procedure for Tietze's syndrome. The researchers followed nine patients with Tietze's syndrome and were able to show improvement in the condition after an injection of steroids.

- *Blood tests.* A sedimentation rate or C-reactive protein test can detect inflammation in Tietze's which would be absent with costochondritis.

- MRI (Magnetic resonance imaging) can also be used to diagnose Tietze's syndrome. It's an excellent way to diagnose both bone and cartilage disorders.

Research published in the May-Jun 2009 issue of Clinical Experimental Rheumatology had a surprising conclusion: a combination of X-ray, CT, MRI and nuclear medicine is the best way to diagnose the disease and rule out other disorders.

The team of Italian researchers evaluated 30 patients with Tietze's syndrome, SAPHO syndrome, ankylosing spondylitis and other costal joint disorders. Each test, the researchers found, gave only a partial clue as to the true nature of the disease. Surprisingly, no one test came out on top.

The idea of multiple tests doesn't completely go against past research in this area. For the past decade or two there has been a lot of debate about which test is the best. Many researchers favor one technique, and three techniques are heralded as "the best" by at least one researcher.

Multiple tests make sense to diagnose Tietze's Syndrome, but there are risks and benefits with every diagnostic tool–including financial constraints. My advice? Find an excellent rheumatologist at a teaching hospital (an MD PhD)–they should be up on current research and will better be able to advise you on current thinking as it crops up. This is especially true with a newly researched disease like Tietze's syndrome.

It's clear from the research that there isn't just one way to diagnose Tietze's syndrome, but what *is* clear is that you should have at least one diagnostic imaging technique done to rule out other causes of your bone pain and swelling. The odds of your Tietze's syndrome being a tumor or skeletal tuberculosis might be small, but no one should suffer the anguish of not knowing exactly what is causing the pain. Insist that your doctor order one of the tests (an ultrasound can often be done in-office), and get peace of mind.

Chapter Five: Treatments

Here are the most commonly recommended treatments for Tietze's syndrome.

- *Rest.* Being barely able to move for six weeks due to Tietze's syndrome was incredibly hard for me—I was a very active person and walked several miles a day. However, avoiding many "normal" activities were a must, to allow my ribs to heal. These included: coughing, heavy breathing (i.e. no intense exercise), lifting, pulling, pushing, repetitive motions (tennis, baseball, scrubbing floors etc.), sneezing, straining, lying down on my back (I slept propped up with many pillows). Lying on my back forced pressure onto my breastbone.

- *Anti-inflammatory drugs.* Nonsteroidal Anti-inflammatory Drugs (NSAIDS) like ibuprofen can help with pain management, but it's important to realize that if your Tietze's syndrome lasts more than a few weeks, you should probably consider alternate therapies. Many painkillers are harsh on the stomach, and are not without side effects. Phenylbutazone used to be indicated for the treatment of Tietze's syndrome, but is no longer sold in the United States for human consumption.

- *Physical therapy.* Physical therapy can be helpful to identify what causes your Tietze's syndrome pain, and to find ways to avoid or reduce the pain. Physical therapists can also help you design a program to strengthen certain muscle groups, so that less stress is placed on the chest area when performing certain tasks. Some physical therapists might use biofeedback when treating Tietze's syndrome.

- *Biofeedback.* Closely related to psychotherapy, biofeedback trains a patient to respond to signals from their body. It has been successful with some stroke patients in regaining use of paralyzed muscles. It works for a myriad of diseases, and it could work for Tietze's syndrome.

- *Ice packs or heat.* I used a heating pad for almost fifteen years for my Tietze's syndrome. I've read elsewhere that variation of hot or cold remedies also work. Some suggestions to try: Heating Pad, Whirlpool bath,

Microwaved, moist towel, Ice, Vapocoolant spray, over-the-counter Heat or Cooling Patches.

- *Prescription patches.* There are many types of prescription pain patches for Tietze's syndrome, including ones that contain lidocaine (an anesthetic) and ibuprofen (a pain reliever which reduces swelling). I tried a prescription patch with ibuprofen for a short time because I didn't want to orally consume a lot of pain medication; it worked very well.

- *TENS (transcutaneous electrical stimulation).* I used a TENS machine during my first and second labors. A TENS machine delivers small electrical pulses to the skin. It doesn't stop intense pain, but it can be useful to stop the mild to moderate pain associated with later-stage Tietze's syndrome. The downside is they are expensive to purchase or rent, and they only work when the machine is on and the pads are applied (in other words, it would be difficult to use it outside of the house).

- *Acupuncture and Electroacupuncture.* I personally have never tried acupuncture, but some people swear by it. Electroacupunture is acupuncture which delivers small electrical pulses to the skin. There's no real scientific evidence that it works for Tietze's syndrome, but as with all alternate therapies—if you think it might help relieve your pain, it could be worth a shot.

- *Massage Therapy.* There's no doubt about it, poor posture and stress can make the symptoms of Tietze's syndrome worse. And it's a vicious cycle: the pain of Tietze's can lead to tense muscles and poor posture. Massage therapy can aid in relaxation—an important part of dealing with the disorder. The more relaxed you are, there less likely you are to tense the muscles around your chest. Plus, people who are relaxed are more inclined to breathe deeply through the stomach (the type of breathing that is most beneficial for Tietze's syndrome).

- *Calcitonin.* Some research has shown that just a small amount of human calcitonin (a drug more commonly used to treat bone loss in postmenopausal women) improved Tietze's syndrome patient's pain after a few days of treatment. According to Ricevuti, the hormone probably works because of the drug's benefit on the immune system and because of its pain-relieving effects.

- *Surgery.* Surgery is usually deemed necessary only for cases of Tietze's syndrome that do not respond to conventional therapy. The surgeon can remove the affected joint.

- *Cortisone injections.* Cortisone shots into the cartilage can temporarily relive pain. These shots do have some side effects (such as temporary pain at the injection site). I had a cortisone shot, and it did a remarkable job at reducing the pain I experienced. An Intercostal nerve block is a steroid injected around the intercostal nerves located under each rib. One of the pain relief methods of last resort, an intercostal nerve block might help with Tietze's syndrome pain if all other methods have been exhausted.

- *Local Anesthetic Injection.* A local anesthetic injection (sometimes in combination with a steroid) can be successful in reducing pain in the vast majority of Tietze's syndrome patients; some reports state it can be up to 97% effective.

- *Stellate Ganglion Block therapy.* I recently came across an article in the Japanese Journal of Anesthesia. The article describes a patient who had severe Tietze's syndrome for more than six years. Her pain (on a scale from 1 to 10) was a full 10; anyone who has ever had Tietze's syndrome knows that kind of pain. But after this specific kind of therapy, the woman's pain diminished to 3 out of 10. The researchers treated the 45-year old patient with SGB therapy. When the woman first arrived, she had the classic signs of Tietze's syndrome-- excruciating pain radiating toward her left shoulder and swelling of one costal cartilage. The researchers performed an ultrasound and saw that the first costal cartilage was swollen. The stellate ganglion is found at the 7th cervical vertebrae, just behind the first rib. Stellate ganglion blocks (injections of local anesthetic) around this area have been shown in the past to help with the pain caused by other chronic diseases, such as complex regional pain syndrome.

The stellate ganglion is also a site targeted in acupuncture to alleviate pain. The researchers injected 5ml of mepivacaine (a local anesthetic) into the stellate ganglion, which reduced the Tietze's syndrome pain for six hours. After the fifth injection (she received one per week), her pain had been reduced to 3 out of 10, and she was able to sleep through the night. Stellate ganglion blocks are known to have this effect--the more you have of them, the longer the pain relief lasts. Stellate ganglion block to treat Tietze's syndrome is performed under local anesthesia and only takes a few minutes. Side effects are rare.

- *Sulfasalazine.*

I'd never heard of sulfasalazine until I read an article in the Journal of Rheumatology on the management of costochondritis (for treatment purposes, both disease can be treated similarly). That's why reading about a possible "new" treatment for Tietze's syndrome was exciting!

The study reported how 11 out of 13 patients initially treated with corticosteroid injections reported recurring symptoms. They were given sulfasalazine, a anti-inflammatory drug commonly given to treat ulcerative colitis and rheumatoid arthritis. Ten of the patients reported success with decreasing their symptoms and stayed on the drug from between six months and 6 years.

Personally, I won't be trying sulfasalazine (or any other prescription drug for my Tietze's syndrome). I've avoided prescription drugs ever since I tried **Vioxx** a decade ago (for those of you unfamiliar with the Vioxx fiasco, it was withdrawn from the market after studies showed serious heart-related side effect). A recent stress test confirmed all is well with my heart but there's still a voice in my head that tells me I had a very close call and I don't want that kind of stress again! I've learned to manage my Tietze's syndrome in other ways, including dietary changes and wearing sports bras. My pain is practically non-existent now, but I remember those years when the pain was excruciating!

Chapter Six: Diet

Tietze noticed that the syndrome caused damage to the cartilage similar to bone disease related to nutrition. Researcher Imamura has since confirmed that malnutrition may also play a role in Tietze's syndrome. Some aspects of diet have been shown to improve the condition.

A couple of years ago a friend of mine recommended I take glucosamine and chondroitin sulfate because it "repairs cartilage damage." He was a runner, and swore by it, although he's never had any major cartilage issues. I purchased a month's supply for $20 and it did precisely nothing. Other supplements recommended by various people over the web include ginger root, evening primrose oil, and bromelain. But do any of these supplements work, or would I be wasting more money? I decided to do a little research before I purchased this time!

Most of the results came from arthritis studies, but like Tietze's syndrome, arthritis involves joints, and inflammation (arthritis literally means "inflamed joints").

Supplements: What Works

- *Willow bark*

The University of Maryland's Complementary Medicine Center states that willow bark is just as effective as aspirin for reducing both pain and inflammation.

- *Ginger root*

According to the University of Maryland, ginger root has been shown to decrease pain in people with arthritis, and is at least as effective as ibuprofen. Considering the lack of side effects of ginger, it seems that ginger root could be a good alternative. Apparently, drinking the tea is just as good as the supplements, and it can also be rubbed into the affected joint.

- *Bromelain, rutosid, and trypsin*

Bromelain by itself has been shown to reduce inflammation. Studies have shown that these three supplements--when taken together for arthritis pain--were as effective as NSAIDS (nonsteroidal anti-inflammatory pills).

- *Vitamin E*

Some sites recommend vitamin E supplements, but the real answer is to eat a balanced diet with nuts, seeds, vegetable oils, and leafy green vegetables. A couple of trials indicated that vitamin e supplements might increase the risk of hemorrhagic stroke, so the best answer is to eat good food!

Supplements: What doesn't work

- *Glucosamine & chondroitin*

Two studies published in the New England Journal of Medicine and Arthritis & Rheumatism revealed that glucosamine alone and chondroitin alone don't fare any better for pain relief on osteoarthritis of the knee (a condition also affecting the body's cartilage) than a placebo (a sugar pill). In combination they might work, but researchers aren't sure. It didn't work for me! On the other hand, it hasn't been shown to cause any harm so it could be worth a try.

- *Omega-3 fatty acid supplements*

Omega-3 fatty acids have been shown in studies to help relieve some symptoms of arthritis, decreasing inflammation in cartilage-containing cells and reducing the activity of enzymes that destroy cells. However, the problem with an omega-3 supplement is that omega-3 fatty acids need to far exceed omega-6 fatty acids. This kind of ratio is often seen in Mediterranean diets which are rich in nuts, fruits, vegetables, and red wine.

If you eat a typical American diet of meat, processed and fried food, an omega-3 supplement will not help you. The key is to eat a balanced healthy diet with better omega-3 to omega-6 ratios. Omega-3 oils can be found in high concentrations in English walnuts, canola oil, soybean oil, flaxseed/linseed oil, and olive oil.

- *Evening primrose oil*

The National Center for Complementary and Alternative Medicine states that evening primrose oil might work. However, the studies that have been done have been small, with design flaws, providing varying results.

Why Vegetarianism Works for Tietze's Syndrome

After going on a vegetarian diet my (sometimes excruciating) symptoms have disappeared after sixteen years of suffering.

I started cooking with the recipes from *The Reactive Hypoglycemia Cookbook*. Nine months later, I haven't had so much as a twinge in my chest. I am convinced it's because of the vegetarian diet. There is an abundance of scientific evidence I have since come across that explains the "miracle" (which in all honesty wasn't so much a miracle as a stroke of luck in eating the right foods).

A lot of research backs up my finding that a vegan diet (rich in fruits, vegetables and soy—*no* sugar, high fructose corn syrup or other artificial additives) can help with the arthritic-like pain of Tietze's Syndrome (arthritis literally means "inflammation of the joints"; Tietze's syndrome usually involves the inflammation of one joint) .

A quick search on Google for food-related arthritic conditions will inform you that there are tens of thousands of suspected food triggers, including dairy products (which have been shown to cause many health problems), and some fruits and vegetables, like eggplant. The evidence from most of these sites is anecdotal. A woman from Colorado who suffered from Gout claimed that she recovered when she switched to a meat-free diet. A man from Hawaii with rheumatoid arthritis claimed that once he stopped eating fish, his arthritis disappeared.

However, there is actual science to back up some of the anecdotal claims. Dava Sobel's groundbreaking 1989 book, *Arthritis: What Works*, surveyed a thousand arthritis patients

(Tietze's syndrome is an arthritic-like disease) to find out what was causing their condition to worsen, and what was causing it to get better. Common triggers included: red meat, dairy products, fat, and sugar--items commonly missing from a vegan diet.

A significant article in the Rheumatology Journal found that after following a vegetarian diet, 59% of patients reported a decrease in joint pain after they stopped eating meat, and 45% reported a decrease in symptoms after they stopped ingesting sugar and coffee. This article that appeared in the Scandinavian Journal of Rheumatology found that one of the culprits was dairy protein, not fat (found in all types of milk and milk products).

If you go to the National Institutes of Health and perform a search for Arthritis/Rheumatism/joint pain and diet, you'll find a glut of research showing that changing to a vegan diet, rich in Omega-3s, helps with arthritic conditions. One article's conclusions included the fact that rheumatoid arthritis symptoms diminished after only four weeks on a vegan diet. It stands to reason that if rheumatism can be helped by diet, so can Tietze's syndrome.

Some other studies that you can find on Pubmed:

- A gluten-free vegan diet improves the signs and symptoms of rheumatoid arthritis.

- A raw vegan diet rich in antioxidants and fiber decreases joint stiffness and pain.

- One study showed that fasting followed by a vegetarian diet can improve symptoms.

Why do researchers think that a vegetarian or vegan diet might work with reduction in joint pain found in Tietze's syndrome? Part of the reason is that antioxidants--found in vegetables--neutralize the free radicals which contribute to joint pain. The nutrients found in abundance in vegetables (vitamins C and E), also assist in this process. Meat on the other hand, supplies very little vitamin E, and no vitamin C.

The diet I went on last year to combat my symptoms was an almost raw-vegan diet. It was almost impossible to stick to--I spent hours in the kitchen cooking (although I did feel better). Over the course of months, I added eggs and meat substitutes (like Morningstar Farms products and Quorn). I even found a substitute for fried chicken--one of my pre-diet favorites.

The result was my book, *The Reactive Hypoglycemic Cookbook*, which is the *only* change in my lifestyle I made.

Although the book is for reactive hypoglycemia, by complete coincidence the diet for that disorder is the same as for the one recommended by researchers for joint pain: meat free, high in antioxidants and Omega-3s, low in fat and no dairy or sugar. After sixteen years of Tietze's syndrome agony, I'm now symptom free. Although I didn't start out liking the idea of going almost-vegan, being pain free has made me a fan...I'd recommend a vegan diet to anyone trying to combat this painful disorder.

Chapter Seven: Selected Recipes

If you don't know where to start with vegetarian meals, here are some simple and nutritious meals to start with.

Portabella Mushroom Burgers

2	ea	garlic clove, chopped		4	ea	Portobello mushroom caps
6	Tbsp	olive oil		4	ea	whole grain or sprouted grain burger buns
½	tsp	thyme				
2	Tbsp	balsamic vinegar				
1	pinch	salt		1	Tbsp	capers, finely chopped
1	pinch	black pepper		¼	cup	Vegenaise spread or Nayonaise spread
				1	ea	tomato
				4	ea	romaine lettuce leaves

Procedure

1. Preheat broiler.
2. Whisk together garlic, olive oil, thyme, vinegar, salt, and pepper.
3. Rinse mushroom caps. Place mushrooms under broiler in a broiler pan.
4. Baste mushrooms with ½ the liquid. Broil for 5 minutes.
5. Turn mushrooms over, baste with remaining liquid. Broil for 5 minutes. Place buns under broiler in last 2 minutes and broil 1 min each side.
6. Mix mayonnaise and capers.
7. Assemble burger, bun, dressing and fixings.

Servings: 4
Yield: 4 burgers

Preparation Time: 20 minutes

Avocado Chik'n Burger

1	Quorn or Morningstar Farms Chik'n Burger	1 to 2	dark green lettuce leaves
1	Ezekiel 4:9 Sprouted Grain burger bun	1	tomato slice
	Vegenaise to taste	1 to 2	slices red onion
		2	slices fresh avocado

Procedure

1. Microwave burgers for 1-2 mins.
2. Toast bun in toaster.
3. Assemble with fixings.

Servings: 1

Nacho Salad

		For guacamole:	2	Tbsp	lemon juice
1	small	avocado			For nachos:
1 ½ cups		silken tofu, soft	3	cups	baked, whole-grain tortilla chips
¼	tsp	salt			
1	pinch	black pepper	4	cups	iceburg lettuce, shredded
1	pinch	cayenne pepper			
¼	tsp	garlic clove, minced	1	can	black beans, drained
			1	cup	Mexican blend shredded cheese
⅛		tsp cumin			
			1 ½	cups	salsa
			4	ea	scallions, chopped

Procedure

1. Place guacamole ingredients in blender. Blend for 3-4 minutes until creamy.
2. In a serving bowl, layer the chips, lettuce, beans, cheese, salsa, and scallions. Top with the guacamole and serve.

Servings: 4
Yield: 8 cups

Egg Salad Sandwich

2	free-range or cage-free eggs	1	pinch salt
1	Tbsp sour cream	¼	cup celery chopped
2	tsp pickle relish	2	slices whole-grain or sprouted-grain bread
2	tsp mayonnaise	1	pinch paprika
¼	tsp mustard		

Procedure

1. Bring eggs to boil in pan of water. Boil for 10 minutes. Cool.
2. In a small bowl, mash all ingredients together.
3. Spread the mixture between two slices of whole-grain bread.

Servings: 2
Yield: 1 full sandwich

Cheese Quesadilla

olive oil spray
1 ea whole wheat tortilla
⅛ cup Mexican blend shredded cheese
½ cup fresh salsa

Procedure

1. Lightly spray a frying pan with oil. Place quesadilla in warmed pan. Sprinkle cheese on and fold over.
2. Cook for 2-3 minutes each side until crispy and cheese has melted. Serve with salsa.

Servings: 1
Yield: 1 quesadilla

10-minute Burger with Mustard Sauce

A quick burger that will satisfy you at the times when you don't feel like cooking.

- 1 ea whole grain or sprouted grain burger bun
- 1 ea vegetarian burger, frozen (try Morningstar Farms)
- 1 tsp honey mustard
- 2 Tbsp Vegenaise spread or Nayonaise spread
- 2 slices tomato
- 2 slices avocado

Procedure

1. Toast bun. Microwave burger according to package directions.
2. Mix honey mustard and Vegenaise. Assemble burger and fixings. Top burger with honey mustard sauce before putting top bun on.

Servings: 1
Yield: 1 burger

Preparation Time: 10 minutes
Cooking Time: 5 minutes

Falafel Sandwich

1 (15-ounce) can regular-sodium chickpeas, drained	4 Ezekiel 4:9 Prophet's pocket bread or other whole grain pita bread
1 pack Casbah Falafel mix	1 cup of Greek yoghurt
1 cloves garlic, minced	½ tsp salt
1 ½ Tbsp chopped fresh cilantro	1 Tbsp lemon juice
	1 Tbsp minced garlic.
	Chopped lettuce, tomatoes, and cucumbers

Procedure

1. Make Falafel mix according to package directions.
2. Mash chickpeas and add garlic. Mix well.
3. Deep fry falafel balls until golden brown.
4. Serve in pita pocket with garnishes and 2T cucumber sauce.

Cucumber Sauce

Grate 1 cucumber and add to 1 cup of Greek yoghurt, ½ tsp salt, 1T lemon juice and 1T minced garlic. Mix well.

Servings: 8

Easy Sweet Potato Chili Fries

12 sweet potato fries (frozen)

1 tablespoon olive oil

½ teaspoon paprika

½ teaspoon garlic powder

½ teaspoon chili powder

½ teaspoon onion powder

Procedure

1. Add all ingredients to a Ziplock bag and shake. Bake fries according to package directions.

Servings: 1

Grilled Quesadilla

1	corn tortilla	2 Tbsp	chopped onion
	Olive oil cooking spray	1	Roma tomato, chopped
½ cup	vegetarian refried beans, can (in Mexican section of grocery store)	1 Tbsp	sour cream
			Salsa
1 oz	Mexican grated cheese blend		

Procedure

1. Spray skillet with cooking spray.
2. Place tortilla on skillet. Top with cheese, onion and tomato.
3. Cook for 1 minute. Fold in half, and cook for additional 1-2 minutes each side until tortilla is brown and filling is bubbling.
4. Serve with refried beans, sour cream, and salsa.

Servings: 1

Southern Fried Popcorn Chik'n

1 tsp. salt

½ tsp. onion powder

1 pinch pepper

1 tsp paprika

1 tsp garlic powder

1 cup unbleached white flour

1 cup wholewheat flour

3 Tbsp yellow mustard

½ cup water

2 Tbsp. baking powder

1 bag. Quorn Chik'n chunks

4 cups olive oil

Procedure

1. Mix salt, onion powder, pepper, paprika, garlic powder, and flour in a large bowl.
2. Defrost Quorn in microwave for about 10 minutes.
3. Mix mustard and water together in a large bowl. Add ½ of flour mixture to bowl and stir well.
4. Place Quorn Chik'n chunks in mustard bowl and mix well until coated.
5. Place about ¼ of the Quorn into the flour & toss well, ensuring all sides covered.
6. Deep fry in olive oil until crispy and brown, about 3-4 minutes. Repeat for remaining product.

Tofurky, Cheese, and Apple Sandwich

2 Slices Tofurky	2 slices English or Irish cheddar
1 Slice Ezekiel 4:9 Sprouted Grain bread	¼ apple, thinly sliced
Vegenaise to taste	

Procedure

1. Assemble sandwich, and enjoy with a serving of fruit and some sweet potato chili fries.

Red Pepper Hummus

1 (16 ounce) can garbanzo beans, drained and rinsed

1 Tbsp olive oil

1 medium red bell pepper, cut into ½ inch pieces

1 Tbsp tahini

1 fresh lime, juiced

1 ½ Tbsp water

½ tsp salt

¼ tsp ground black pepper

¼ tsp garlic powder

Procedure

1. Combine all the ingredients in a blender, and blend on high until smooth and creamy, 1 to 2 minutes. Will keep in the refrigerator for up to 3 days. Serve with baked pita chips, carrots, celery, and/or red pepper strips.

Servings: 10

Spicy Bean Burgers

1 can black beans, drained

½ green bell pepper, chopped finely

½ onion, chopped finely

3 cloves garlic, minced

1 free range egg

1 Tbsp chili powder

1 Tbsp cumin

1 t chili sauce

½ cup breadcrumbs, made from placing 2 slices torn Ezekiel 4:9 into a blender

Procedure

Combine all the ingredients in a bowl. Add breadcrumbs until you can easily form a ball. Flatten into a patty, and fry in olive oil 2-3 minutes each side, until crispy. Serve with a salad, or in an Ezekiel 4:9 burger bun with burger fixings.

Mexico City Omelet

4 free range eggs	¼ cup chopped red pepper
⅛ cup soy milk	¼ cup chopped fresh tomato
Pinch salt	¼ cup chopped onion
Pinch pepper	¼ cup black beans
	¼ cup vegan cheese shreds
	Olive oil spray
	Fresh, coarsely chopped salsa

Procedure

3. Whisk eggs, salt, pepper, and soy milk together.
4. Spray a griddle with olive oil. Fry pepper and onion for 2-3 minutes. Add tomato, cook an additional 1 minute. Move to side of griddle.
5. Respray griddle. Pour ½ of egg mixture and cook until almost done. Flip. Add ½ of vegetable mixture to center of omelet with ⅛ cup vegan cheese. Fold omelet over in half.
6. Cook omelet for 1 min each side.
7. Serve with salsa.

Yield: 2 omelets

Minestrone Soup

- ⅓ cup whole-grain macaroni
- 1 tsp extra-virgin olive oil
- ⅓ cup diced onion
- 4 cups water
- 1 cup frozen carrot pieces
- ⅓ cup ½-inch celery pieces
- 1 cup ¼-inch zucchini pieces
- 1 cup diced canned tomatoes
- 1 cup low-sodium canned kidney beans, drained
- 1 ½ tsp McKay's Beef-Style Instant Broth and Seasoning
- 1 tsp salt
- 1 tsp dried basil
- ½ tsp dried oregano
- ⅛ tsp garlic powder
- 1 bay leaf

Procedure

1. Place all ingredients in a slow cooker and cook for 8 hours on low.

Servings: 7

Spicy Marinara Sauce

1 can chopped tomatoes	2 Tbsp Italian seasoning (in herb & spices)
½ pint cherry tomatoes	
½ cup frozen mixed peppers	2 basil leaves
3 Tbsp Emeril's Bayou Blast seasoning	1 tsp dried oregano

Procedure

1. Place all ingredients in a slow cooker. Cook on low for 8 hours.

Servings: 8

Ten Vegetable Soup

4 cups water	1 pinch Italian seasoning
1 ⅓ cups cubed unpeeled red potatoes	½ tsp dried thyme
1 cup sliced yellow squash	3 tsp McKay's Chicken-Style Instant Broth and Seasoning
1 can chopped tomatoes	1 tsp salt
⅔ cup sliced celery	2 tsp nutritional yeast flakes
1 ⅓ cups sliced carrots	⅓ cup fresh spinach
⅔ cup chopped onion	⅓ cup frozen green beans
1 bay leaf	⅓ cup frozen green peas
½ tsp garlic powder	2 Tbsp chopped fresh parsley
1 tsp onion powder	

Procedure

10. Combine all ingredients in a slow cooker. Cook on low for 8 hours.

Servings: 8

Spicy Slow Cooker Chili

1 bag Quorn or other meatless crumbles (i.e. Morningstar farm)

32 oz tomato juice (approx ⅔ of a 46 fl. oz. bottle)

1 can tomato sauce

1 ⅔ cup chopped onion

½ cup celery, chopped

¼ cup green pepper, chopped

¼ cup red pepper, chopped

½ cup chili powder

2 tsp cumin

1 ½ tsp garlic powder

1 tsp salt

½ tsp black pepper

½ tsp oregano

½ tsp cayenne pepper

2 cups chili or kidney beans

Procedure

1. Place all ingredients in a slow cooker. Cook on low for 8 hours.

Servings: 6

Spicy Quinoa Soup

1	Tbsp extra-virgin olive oil	1	can diced tomatoes
½	cup quinoa, rinsed and patted dry	½	cup frozen whole-kernel yellow corn
2 ½ tsp	ground cumin seed	1	tsp salt
1	tsp ground dried thyme	7	cups low-sodium vegetable broth
1	tsp dried oregano leaves		
2	whole cloves	1 ¾ cups	black beans, drained
¼	cup chopped onion	2	Tbsp chopped fresh cilantro leaves
1	cup chopped red bell pepper		
2	cloves garlic, minced		
1	jalapeño chili, seeds removed, minced		

Procedure

1. Add all ingredients to a slow cooker, and cook on low for 8 hours.

Servings: 8

Southwest Soup

1	tsp extra-virgin olive oil	7	cups quartered fresh Roma tomatoes
½	cup diced onion		
¾	cup julienned carrot	1	cup water
⅓	cup thinly sliced celery	½	cup frozen whole-kernel yellow corn
¼	cup diced yellow squash		
1	tsp McKay's Beef-Style Instant Broth and Seasoning	½	can black beans
		1	tsp salt
		¼	cup chopped fresh cilantro

Procedure

1. Add ingredients to slow cooker. Cook on low for 8 hours.

Servings: 6

Black Bean Soup

2 cans black beans

1 ½ quarts water

1 carrot, chopped

½ cup celery, chopped

1 red onion, chopped

6 Tbsp minced garlic

2 green bell peppers, chopped

2 jalapenos, seeded and minced

¼ cup dry lentils

1 (28 ounce) can peeled and diced tomatoes

2 Tbsp chili powder

2 tsp ground cumin

½ tsp dried oregano

½ tsp ground black pepper

3 Tbsp red wine vinegar

1 Tbsp salt

½ cup uncooked brown rice

Procedure

Place all ingredients in a slow cooker. Cook on low for 6 hours.

Servings: 6

Chik'n Kofta Curry

1 lb Quorn Chik'n chunks	¼ cup tomato puree
3 onions, chopped	½ tsp turmeric powder
½ tsp chili powder	3 green peppers, chopped
2 cups coconut milk	1 tsp chopped cilantro
2 tsp minced ginger	1 tsp chopped garlic
	2 tsp Garam masala

Procedure

15. Place all ingredients except for coconut milk into a slow cooker. Cook on low for 8 hours. Add coconut milk, blend and cook on low for 30 minutes.

Meatballs and Pasta

1 pack vegan or vegetarian meatballs

⅛ tsp dried basil

1 Tbsp Emeril's Bayou Blast

1 can chopped tomatoes, Italian style

1 Tbsp fresh oregano

1 jar marinara sauce

1 package whole grain spaghetti noodles

Grated parmesan cheese

Procedure

Place all ingredients in a slow cooker. Cook on low for 8 hours. Cook spaghetti according to package directions.

Servings: 6

Indian Lentil Soup

- 1 cup red lentils
- 5 cups water
- 1 clove garlic, crushed
- 1 Tbsp extra-virgin olive oil
- 1 cup chopped onion
- ½ cup thinly sliced celery
- 1 cup finely diced carrots
- 1 ½ Tbsp tomato paste
- 1 bay leaf
- ⅛ tsp chili powder
- 1 ½ tsp salt
- 1 ½ cups canned whole crushed tomatoes
- ½ cup chopped fresh parsley

Procedure

1. Place all ingredients in slow cooker. Cook on low for 8 hours.

Servings: 8

Eggplant Curry

1 large eggplant

2 Tbsp vegetable oil

1 Tbsp cumin seeds

1 onion, chopped

1 Tbsp ginger paste

1 Tbsp garlic

1 Tbsp curry powder

1 tsp dried cilantro

1 tomato, diced

½ cup plain soy yogurt

1 fresh jalapeno, finely chopped

1 tsp salt

4 Tbsp cilantro, finely chopped

Procedure

Place all ingredients except yoghurt and cilantro in slow cooker. Cook on low for 7-8 hours. Add yoghurt 10 minutes before serving, stirring well. Garnish with cilantro.

Chik'n Noodle Soup

1 ½ tsp extra-virgin olive oil	3 ½ cups water
½ cup chopped onion	1 cup uncooked whole grain pasta
1 clove garlic, minced	
¼ cup minced carrot	1 cup Quorn Chik'n chunks, cut into ¼ inch pieces
3 Tbsp McKay's Chicken-Style Instant Broth and Seasoning	½ cup low-sodium canned diced tomatoes
	1 Tbsp dried parsley

Procedure

Place all ingredients in a slow cooker. Cook on low for 8 hours.

Servings: 6

Cream of Celery Soup

2 ½	cups	water	4	cups	½-inch celery pieces
1	tsp	McKay's Beef-Style Instant Broth and Seasoning	2	Tbsp	cornstarch
			2	cups	unsweetened or plain soymilk
1	tsp	McKay's Chicken-Style Instant Broth and Seasoning	¼	tsp	dried marjoram
			1 ½	Tbsp	low sodium soy sauce
1	cup	diced, peeled red potato	1	tsp	salt
			1 pinch	tsp	cayenne pepper
1	cup	sliced onion			
½	cup	chopped celery			

Procedure

Combine in a slow cooker. Cook on low for 8 hours.

Servings: 8

Indian Curried Chick Peas

1 Tbsp canola oil	½ jalapeño chili, seeds removed, and finely diced
½ cup water	
1 tsp cumin seed	
1 ½ cups finely chopped onions	1 tsp Indian curry powder
	1 tsp salt
2 cloves garlic, minced	½ cup reduced-fat coconut milk
1 (14.5-ounce) can crushed tomatoes	
	¼ cup chopped fresh cilantro
2 (15-ounce) cans regular-sodium chickpeas, drained (3 cups)	

Procedure

Add all ingredients except for coconut milk into a slow cooker. Cook on low for 7 hours. Add coconut milk, cook on low for additional 1 hour.

Servings: 8

Harvest Soup

- 5 cups 1-inch cubes squash, zucchini, or other fall vegetables
- 1 cup diced celery
- ½ cup diced onion
- 4 cups water
- 1 Tbsp McKay's Chicken-Style Instant Broth and Seasoning
- ½ tsp salt
- 1 pinch tsp cayenne pepper

Procedure

Place all the ingredients into a slow cooker. Cook on low for 8 hours.

Servings: 7

Tomato Quiche

This bakes more like a thick crust pie than a quiche. However, even my finicky ten-year-old gave this dish the thumbs up! If you prefer, substitute mushrooms or onions (or a combination) in place of the tomatoes.

- 1 cup whole wheat bread crumbs
- ¼ cup whole wheat flour
- ½ cup bulgur or cracked wheat
- ½ cup Toasted Oats
- ¼ tsp salt
- ¾ tsp marjoram
- ½ cup vegan buttery spread, melted
- 1 Tbsp olive oil
- 1 ea sliced tomato (large)
- ½ tsp thyme
- ¼ lb sharp cheddar, grated
- 2 ea eggs
- ⅛ cup egg whites (try Organic Valley)
- 1 cup soy milk
- ½ tsp paprika

Procedure

1. Preheat oven to 350 degrees. Mix whole wheat bread crumbs, whole wheat flour, bulgur wheat, salt, toasted oats, and ¼ tsp of the marjoram, together in a large bowl. Add buttery spread and mix well.
2. Press into a 8" pie dish. Bake for 10 minutes.
3. Sprinkle grated cheddar over crust.
4. Saute mushrooms, scallions, thyme, and oregano in olive oil for 3 minutes until softened. Pour evenly into pie.
5. Whisk eggs, egg white, and milk. Pour over mushrooms.
6. Top with sprinkled paprika.
7. Bake at 375 degrees for 40 minutes until golden brown.

Servings: 8
Yield: 1 quiche

Andrew's Veggie Lasagna

My fourteen-year-old son made this dish for a Friday night supper with friends. It was such a hit, even my friends wanted the recipe!

6	ea	whole wheat lasagna noodles
2	Tbsp	olive oil
½	cup	onion, finely chopped
1	ea	garlic clove, minced
1	tsp	oregano, fresh
2	tsp	basil, fresh
½	tsp	black pepper
1	cup	zucchini, diced
1	cup	mushrooms, diced
3	cups	spinach

For Ricotta Filling:

6	ea	Roma tomato, chopped
1	lb	firm tofu
⅛	cup	lemon juice
2	tsp	xylitol
½	tsp	salt
2	tsp	basil
2	Tbsp	olive oil
½	tsp	garlic clove, minced

Procedure

1. Cook noodles according to package directions.
2. Stir fry onion and garlic in olive oil for 4 minutes until softened.
3. Puree tomatoes in a blender. Add to onion and garlic. Add oregano, basil, pepper, zucchini, mushrooms, and spinach. Simmer for 10 minutes.
4. Place Ricotta filling ingredients in a large bowl and mash well.

5. Spray a 13" x 9" lasagna pan with cooking spray. Place ⅓ of the marinara sauce on the bottom of the pan. Cover with 3 noodles and ½ the ricotta cheese. Repeat. Top with marinara sauce.
6. Bake for 45 minutes.

Servings: 6

Oven Temperature: 350°F

Preparation Time: 30 minutes

Black Bean Enchiladas

1 (8-ounce) can tomato sauce	1 tsp dry onion soup mix
½ cup water	½ cup low-sodium canned black beans, drained
⅛ tsp ground cumin	
3 Tbsp picante sauce	¼ cup finely chopped onion
1 ½ tsp chili powder	2 Tbsp chopped fresh cilantro
½ (12-ounce) meatless burger crumbles	
	½ cup Vegan Cheese Sauce (see recipe)
	6 Food for Life Sprouted Corn tortillas
	½ bag vegan grated cheese

Procedure

7. Stir the tomato sauce, water, cumin, salsa, and chili powder together in a medium saucepan. Heat through and simmer for 5 minutes.
8. Add the crumbles and heat for an additional 5 minutes.
9. Add onion soup mix, beans, onion, cilantro, and ¼ cup of cheese sauce. Mix well.
10. Preheat oven to 350°F.
11. Place the tortillas in a microwave for 15-20 seconds to soften.

12. Divide the filling and fill each tortilla, folding the tortilla underneath.
13. Pour cheese sauce on top of enchiladas.
14. Top with vegan grated cheese.
15. Bake for 15 minutes until the cheese has melted and the enchiladas are heated through.

Servings: 6

Vegan Cheese Sauce

1 ¼ cups water

¼ cup raw cashew pieces

1 Tbsp nutritional yeast flakes

1 cup frozen, cooked brown rice

1 tsp salt

¼ tsp garlic powder

1 tsp onion powder

1 ½ Tbsp lemon juice

Procedure

1. Blend all the ingredients in a food processor or blender until creamy, about 5 minutes.

Servings: 8

Strawberry-Poppy Seed Salad

1 head romaine lettuce - rinsed, dried, and chopped

1 pint fresh strawberries, sliced

1 sweet onion, sliced

½ cup Vegenaise

2 tablespoons red wine vinegar

⅓ cup fructose

¼ cup milk

2 tablespoons poppy seeds

2 bunches fresh spinach - chopped, washed and dried

Procedure

Combine Vegenaise, vinegar, fructose, milk and poppy seeds until creamy and blended. Combine salad ingredients and toss until evenly coated.

Yield: 6 servings

Eggplant Curry

- 1 lb eggplant, peeled, and cut in ½ " cubes
- 2 Tbsp canola oil
- 2 Tbsp ginger
- 3 ea jalapeño chili, seeds removed, and finely diced
- 4 tsp ground cumin
- 2 ea onion, chopped
- 2 ea garlic clove, minced
- ⅛ tsp red chili pepper (cayenne)
- 1 tsp garam masala
- 4 ea Roma tomato, chopped
- ¼ tsp turmeric powder
- 1 pinch salt
- 4 Tbsp cilantro
- ½ cup cashews
- 1 cup brown rice, cooked
- 2 ea naan, wholewheat

Procedure

1. Place cubed eggplant in a baking pan. Spray with olive oil for 1-2 seconds. Broil for 8 minutes, until flesh is soft.
2. Stir fry jalapeno, ginger, and cumin in the canola oil for 1 minute.
3. Add onion and garlic to the pan. Stir fry 2-3 minutes until onions are softened.
4. Add chili pepper, turmeric, salt, tomatoes and cooked eggplant to pan
5. Simmer for 15 minutes on low to allow flavors to blend.
6. Top with chopped cilantro and cashews. Serve with naan bread.

Servings: 4
Yield: 4 servings

Spinach Lasagna Rolls

14	whole grain lasagna noodles	4	cups chopped fresh spinach
4	cups water-packed, extra-firm tofu, drained	2	Tbsp dried basil leaves
		2	tsp dried oregano leaves
½ cup	unsweetened soymilk	2	Tbsp nutritional yeast flakes
2 tsp	fresh lemon juice		
1 cup	finely chopped onion	1 ½ tsp	salt
8	cloves garlic, minced	1 jar marinara Sauce	
		1 cup mozzarella cheese	

Procedure

1. Preheat oven to 350 degrees.
2. Cook lasagna according to package directions until al dente.
3. Blend tofu, soymilk, and lemon juice in a blender for 1 minute.
4. Sauté onion and garlic in 1 Tbsp water for 2-3 minutes until softened. Add spinach and sauté for 2-3 minutes, until spinach has softened.
5. Stir in basil, oregano, nutritional yeast flakes, and salt.
6. Divide mixture into 14. Place one portion into a lasagna noodle, roll up and place in greased 9"x13" baking dish.
7. Pour marinara sauce mixture over lasagna rolls.

14. Sprinkle with mozzarella cheese. Bake, covered for 30 minutes. Uncover and bake for an additional 10 minutes.

Servings: 14

Caesar Salad

6 cups chopped romaine lettuce	1 cup organic, vegan croutons
½ cup thinly sliced red onion	½ cup Caesar Salad Dressing (see recipe)
¼ cup pitted black olives	

Procedure

15 Place all ingredients except for croutons in a bowl and toss well. Add croutons, and serve.

Servings: 7

Caesar Salad Dressing

½ cup Vegenaise	2 Tbsp nutritional yeast flakes
2 Tbsp canola oil	½ tsp salt
2 Tbsp fresh lemon juice	¼ tsp citric acid
2 cloves garlic, minced	

Procedure

Combine all the ingredients in a small bowl and mix until smooth and creamy.

Servings: 8

Amora's Salsa

- 2 large fresh tomatoes, whole and unpeeled
- 1 can Roma tomatoes, chopped
- 1 Tbsp canned green chilies
- 2 Tbsp diced red onion
- 3 Tbsp finely chopped fresh cilantro
- ¾ tsp salt
- 1 Tbsp lime juice

Procedure

Place all ingredients in a blender and blend for 30 seconds. Serve with baked, whole grain tortilla chips.

Servings: 14

Dill and Cucumber Salad

2	cups ½-inch cucumber cubes	⅛	tsp salt
		⅛	tsp garlic powder
1	cup ½-inch tomato pieces	½	cup sour cream
¼	cup ¼-inch red onion pieces		
½	tsp dried dill weed		

Procedure

Stir the celery seed, dill weed, salt, garlic powder and sour cream together. Add vegetables and toss.

Servings: 7

Grilled Portobello Mushrooms

4	large Portobello mushrooms, de-stemmed and washed	4 Tbsp honey mustard
5	Tbsp light Italian vinaigrette dressing (i.e. Kraft)	

Procedure

19. Preheat broiler to medium-high.
20. Marinate the mushrooms in the vinaigrette for 5 minutes.
21. Broil 4 to 5 minutes each side until hot through.
22. Top each mushroom with honey mustard. Serve immediately.

Yield: 4 Mushrooms

Appendix 1

Web Resources

Tietze's Syndrome Info:
http://www.tietzessyndrome.com

All the latest information and research about Tietze's Syndrome on the web.

The Journal of Alternate and Complementary Medicine:
http://www.liebertonline.com/toc/acm/8/1

Several full text articles from this peer-reviewed journal on alternative medicine topics are available on this website.

PubMed: http://www.pubmed.com

A free search engine for locating articles in the sciences and biomedical fields. Maintained by the United States National Library of Medicine at the National Institutes of Health.

University of Maryland: http://www.umm.edu/altmed/

An index of complementary and alternative medicine, including herbs, supplements, and their usefulness.

BLOGS

Tsetse Syndrome Attack

http://kaishan-sg.blogspot.com/2009/06/tsetse-attack.html

Kai Shan in Singapore blogs about his Tietze Syndrome pain, which he (tongue-in-cheek) calls Tsetse, which is often confused with Tietze's.

My Tietze's Blog

http://mytietzesblog.blogspot.com/

Charlie from England blogs about her Tietze's in an effort to disseminate correct info about Tietze's. A dedicated Tietze's blog.

Standing Silent on Tietzes syndrome

http://community.livejournal.com/costochondrits/2380.html?thread=6476

This blog post by Standing Silent really struck a chord with me. I think it's because when I first got Tietze's, I felt so alone--just like her.

Costochondritis, Tietze's syndrome, and Chronic Fatigue Syndrome

http://cfsandstuff.blogspot.com/2009/03/costochondritis.html

I found this blog by Fiona interesting because of her issues with Chronic Fatigue Syndrome (CFS).

References:

Alvarez, F. et. al. Primary costochondritis due to Escherichia coli Scandinavian Journal of Infectious Disease. 2000;32(4):430-1.

Boehme, M. et al. Tietze's syndrome--a chameleon under the thoracic abdominal pain syndrome Klin Wochenschr. 1988 Nov 15;66(22):1142-5.

Cameron, H. & Fornasier, V. Tietze's disease Journal of. clinical. Pathology., 1974, 27, 960-962.

Caranasi, RJ, Christian JJ, Brindley HH. Costosternal chondrodynia: a variant of Tietze's syndrome? Dis Chest. 1962 May;41:559–562.

Cocco, R. et al. Lymphomas presenting as Tietze's syndrome: a report of 4 clinical cases. Ann Ital Med Int. 1999 Apr-Jun;14(2):118-23.

Fauci, A & Langford, C. (eds.) Harrison's Rheumatology. New York: McGraw-Hill 2006

Freeston J, Karim Z, Lindsay K, And Gough A. Can Early Diagnosis and Management of Costochondritis Reduce Acute Chest Pain Admissions? Retrieved July 16, 2009 from http://www.jrheum.com/subscribers/04/11/2269.html

Frontera, W. & Silver, J. Essentials of Physical Medicine and Rehabilitation. Philadelphia, PA: Saunders Elsevier, 2008.

Gill, G. Epidemic of Tietze's Syndrome. British Medical Journal 1977;2:499 (20 August).

Gill,. A. M.;. Jones,. R. A., and. Pollack,. L.Tietze's Disease. British Medical Journal. 2:155. (Aug. 8). 1942

Guglielmi G, Cascavilla A, Scalzo G, Salaffi F, Grassi W. Imaging of sternocostoclavicular joint in spondyloarthropaties and other rheumatic conditions. Clin Exp Rheumatol. 2009 May-Jun;27(3):402-8

Hafström I, Ringertz B, Spångberg A, von Zweigbergk L, Brannemark S, Nylander I, Rönnelid J, Laasonen L, Klareskog L.Rheumatology (Oxford). 2001 Oct;40(10):1175-9..

Imamura, M. and Imamura, I Essentials of Physical Medicine. Philadelphia, PA: Saunders. 2008.

Krohn-Grimberghe B, et. al. Pleomorphic T-cell lymphoma with chondropathia tuberosa; a case report and review. Anticancer Res. 1999 May-Jun;19(3B):2221-8.

Mansel, R. Recent developments in the study of benign breast disease. New York, NY: Parthenon Publishing Group. 1997.

Martino, G. et al. Tietze's syndrome in the elderly: description of a case and review of the literature. Il Giornale di Chirurgia. 1994 Mar;15(3):119-23.

Marudanayagam, A. Gnanadoss, J. Multifocal Skeletal Tuberculosis: A Report of Three Cases. Iowa Orthopedic Journal. 2006; 26: 151–153

Mathew, A. et. al. Costosternal chondrodynia simulating recurrent breast cancer unveiled by FDG PET. Clinical Nuclear Medicine. 2008 May;33(5):330-2.

McCarty, D. & Koopman, W. Arthritis and allied conditions. NY, New York: Williams & Wilkins. 1993

McDougall, J. et al. Effects of a Very Low-Fat, Vegan Diet in Subjects with Rheumatoid Arthritis. The Journal of Alternative and Complementary Medicine. Volume 8, Number 1, 2002, pp. 71–75

Müller H, de Toledo FW, Resch KL. Fasting followed by vegetarian diet in patients with rheumatoid arthritis: a systematic review. Scandinavian Journal of Rheumatology. 2001;30(1):1-10.

O'Neal, M. Complex strain injury involving an intercostal hematoma in a professional baseball player. Clinical Journal Sport Medicine. 2008 Jul;18(4):372-3.

Pappalardo et. al, Reflexions on the Tietze syndrome. Clinica Terapeutica. 1995 Nov;146(11):675-82.

Pijning, J, et. al. Tietze's syndrome in a 2-year-old boy. Ned Tijdschr Geneeskd . Volume: 147, Issue: 43, Date: 2003 Oct 25, Pages: 2134-6. 2003

Ricevuti G. Effects of human calcitonin on pain in the treatment of Tietze's syndrome Clinical Therapies. 1985;7(6):669-73.

Ruddy S et al (eds.). Kelley's Textbook of Rheumatology, W B Saunders Co, 2000.

Russell, J. et. al. Elevated cerebrospinal fluid levels of substance p in patients with the fibromyalgia syndrome. Arthritis and Rheumatism. Volume 37 Issue 11, Pages 1593 – 1601.

Shiel, W. Costochondritis & Tietze Syndrome. Article posted on website medicinenet.com. Retrieved June 10, 2009 from http://www.medicinenet.com/costochondritis_and_tietze_syndrome/article.htm

Starlanyl, D. Reactive Hypoglycemia (RHG): FMS&MPS Complex Perpetuating Factor. Article posted on website Fibromyalgia Information. Retrieved June 9, 2009 from http://fibromyalgia.ncf.ca/dshypogl.htm.

Sueiro Blanco F, Estévez Schwarz I, Ayán, Cancela JM, and Martín V Potential Benefits of Non-Pharmacologica Cl Therapies in Fibromyalgia. Open Rheumatology Journal. 2008; 2: 1–6.

Tamakawa, S et al. Stellate ganglion block therapy for a patient with Tietze's syndrome. Journal of Anesthesia Springer Japan. Volume 11, Number 3 / September, 1997

Tatelman M, Drouillard EJP. Tuberculosis of the ribs. American Journal of Rheumatology 1953; 70: 923-935.

Thongngarm T, et. al. Malignant tumor with chest wall pain mimicking Tietze's syndrome. Clinical Rheumatology. 2001;20(4):276-8.

Tumakawa, S. Stellate ganglion block therapy for a patient with Tietze's syndrome. Journal of Anesthesia. Volume 11, Number 3 / September, 1997 Japan: Springerlink.

Valtonen, E. Phenylbutazone in the Treatment of Tietze's Disease. Annals of the Rheumatic Diseases 1967;26:133-135

Wright, F. Radiology of The Chest and Related Conditions. New York, NY: Taylor and Francis, 2002.

10-Minute Burger, 47, 57, 65
10-minute Burger with Mustard Sauce, 51
Acupuncture, 31
Alexander Tietze, 6
Andrew's Veggie Lasagna, 78
Anti-inflammatory Drugs (NSAIDS), 29
Arthritis, 20, 39, 41, 42, 99, 100
Baked Falafels, 52
Baked Sweet Potato, 53
Biofeedback, 30
Black Bean Enchiladas, 80
Blood tests., 26
Breast Implants, 23
Butternut Harvest Soup, 76
Caesar Salad, 87
Caesar Salad Dressing, 88
calcitonin, 32
Cancer, 21, 23
Cashew Jack Cheese Sauce, 82
causes, 7, 16, 18, 21, 22, 25, 27, 30
Cheese Quesedilla, 50
Chiapas Salsa, 89
Chickpea Noodle Soup, 73
Chunky Marinara Sauce, 63
Classic Hummus, 58
cortisone, 33
costochondritis, 6, 7, 8, 9, 10, 16, 21, 24, 26, 95, 97, 100
costosternal chondrodynia, 10
Cream of Celery Soup, 74

Crohn's disease, 21
CT scan, 23
Curried Garbanzos, 75
Diet, 37
Dill Cucumber Salad, 90
E-coli, 23
Egg Salad Sandwich, 49
Eggplant Curry, 84
Fibromyalgia, 19, 100, 101
Fiesta Burrito, 61
Garden Minestrone Soup, 62
Grilled Portobello Mushrooms, 91
Grilled Quesadilla, 54, 55
heart attack, 5, 7, 9, 14
ibuprofen, 6, 29, 31, 38
Indian Lentil Soup, 71, 72
local anesthetic, 33, 34
micro trauma, 19
MRI, 15, 23, 26
Nacho Salad, 48
Nut Meatballs, 70
Peanut Butter-Flaxseed Cookies, 83
Phenylbutazone, 30
Physical therapy, 30
Pleomorphic T-cell lymphoma, 13
Portabella Mushroom Burgers, 46
Sautéed Button Mushroom Soup, 69
slipping rib syndrome, 9, 11
Southwest Soup, 67
Spicy Vegetable Quinoa Soup, 66

Spinach Lasagne, 85
Stellate Ganglion Block, 34
Summer Vegetable Soup, 64
Supplements, 38
Surgery, 33
syphilis, 22
TENS, 31

Tofu Egg Salad, 59
Tomato Quiche, 77
Trauma, 19
tumor, 15, 23, 27, 101
Ultrasound, 25
Vioxx, 9
Xeroradiography, 25

LaVergne, TN USA
13 January 2011
212281LV00004B/63/P